SBAs and EMQs in Psychiatry for Medical Students

SBAs and EMQs in Psychiatry for Medical Students

DR NEEL SHARMA

BSc (Hons), MBChB

Foundation Year Two Doctor
Homerton University Hospital NHS Foundation Trust
London

Foreword by

DR TIAGO VILLANUEVA

Past Editor of the *Student BMJ*

Radcliffe Publishing
Oxford • New York

Radcliffe Publishing Ltd
18 Marcham Road
Abingdon
Oxon OX14 1AA
United Kingdom

www.radcliffe-oxford.com
Electronic catalogue and worldwide online ordering facility.

British Library Cataloguing in Publication Data

A catalogue record for this book is available from the British Library.

ISBN-13: 978 184619 414 6

The paper used for the text pages of this book
is FSC certified. FSC (The Forest Stewardship
Council) is an international network to promote
responsible management of the world's forests.

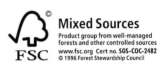

Mixed Sources
Product group from well-managed
forests and other controlled sources
www.fsc.org Cert no. SGS-COC-2482
© 1996 Forest Stewardship Council

FSC

Typeset by Pindar NZ, Auckland, New Zealand
Printed and bound by TJI Digital, Padstow, Cornwall, UK

Contents

Foreword

It is a well-known fact that psychiatry is not any medical student's cup of tea. All contributions to soften and ameliorate a medical student's journey through the convoluted world of psychiatry are very welcome and Dr Neel Sharma's latest book points truly in that direction. If you're looking for a structured and comprehensive framework to enable you to review the complete ins and outs of psychiatry then this book is most definitely for you. Neel Sharma resorts to a clever and balanced mixture of SBAs and EMQs with relevant, concise answers that cater for both review and exam preparation purposes. With a few adaptations, it should definitely be translated into other languages so that students from other countries outside the UK can benefit as well from Neel Sharma's knowledge.

Dr Tiago Villanueva
Past Editor of the *Student BMJ*
November 2009

Preface

As a recent medical graduate I understand all too well the pressures faced during medical school. Lectures, tutorials, never-ending ward rounds, outpatient clinics, course work assignments and, of course, let us not forget the gruelling end-of-year exams. Trying to retain and, more importantly, understand all the common (and not so common) clinical diseases and presentations truly seems an impossible task.

With the advent of the Universities Medical Assessment Partnership (UMAP) there has now been a move away from testing specific clinical facts to an assessment focused on preparing yourself as a foundation doctor and the knowledge such a trainee needs on a daily basis. Currently, 14 UK medical schools are part of UMAP and their exams now require candidates to decide, for example, what would be the most appropriate initial investigation or what management plan they would instigate first when faced with a clinical problem. Hardly an easy task based on the little experience one gains as an undergraduate in such decisions.

This self-assessment book is designed to help students tackle both the new form of assessment as well as the traditional style of examination. Questions covering all common psychiatric presentations are included as SBA and EMQ formats with relevant, concise explanations as answers.

I sincerely hope that this book is of use in preparing for your forthcoming examinations and wish you all the success in your future medical careers.

Neel Sharma
November 2009

Education and work are the levers to uplift a people. Work alone will not do it unless inspired by the right ideals and guided by intelligence.

WEB Du Bois 1868–1963

I would like to dedicate this book to my parents, Ravi and Anita, and my sister Ravnita. Without their continued support and encouragement none of this would have truly been possible.

Useful references

The British Journal of Psychiatry. Available at: http://bjp.rcpsych.org/
Evidence-Based Mental Health. Available at: http://ebmh.bmj.com
Semple D, Smyth R, Burns J, *et al. Oxford Handbook of Psychiatry*.
    Oxford: Oxford University Press; 2005.
The Royal College of Psychiatrists. Available at: www.rcpsych.ac.uk

Questions

Single best answer

1   The following are all features of Schneider's first rank symptoms EXCEPT:

   a Thought broadcast

   b Auditory hallucinations

   c Delusional perception

   d Weight gain

   e Somatic passivity

2   Paranoid schizophrenia is characterised by the following symptoms EXCEPT:

   a Delusions of persecution

   b Delusions of reference

   c Incoherent speech

   d Auditory hallucinations of a threatening nature

   e Delusions of bodily change

3 A 25-year-old cannabis misuser presents to A&E stating that Hulk Hogan has been following her. She is noted to be grimacing excessively and clicks her fingers constantly during the consultation. What is the most likely diagnosis?

    a Paranoid schizophrenia

    b Catatonic schizophrenia

    c Bipolar affective disorder

    d Residual schizophrenia

    e Depression

4 The following are all risk factors associated with the development of schizophrenia EXCEPT:

    a Spring births

    b Winter births

    c Drug misuse

    d Life events

    e Alcohol misuse

5 A middle-aged woman presents to A&E stating that the Mafia want to kill her and that she can hear voices stating that people want to set her bedroom on fire. The following are all likely to be true EXCEPT:

    a She is of a lower socioeconomic class

    b She is not married

    c She is likely to be misusing illicit drugs

    d She is 65 years or over

    e She may have suffered a recent life event

6 A middle-aged woman presents to A&E with her mother stating that she has been physically assaulted by her neighbour. On consultation with her mother you are informed that this is in fact not true. Her mother states that her daughter has been verbally abusive to her neighbour for many months. She also explains that her daughter has been using the internet recently to learn more about the devil and keeps bags of salt in her bath to help cleanse her soul. What is the next most appropriate step in management?

a Citalopram

b Sodium valproate

c Olanzapine

d Fluoxetine

e Lithium

7 A 45-year-old woman with a background history of paranoid schizophrenia is referred to A&E by her general practitioner (GP). Her GP notes that she has been non-compliant with her oral risperidone 4 mg at night for the past two months. During the consultation, the patient discusses her concerns about the rapid advancement of technology and states that technology in her home may destroy buildings and people. On further consultation the patient states that she feels the medication is of no use. Which management plan would you instigate first?

a Electroconvulsive therapy (ECT)

b Cognitive behavioural therapy

c Fluoxetine

d Restart oral risperidone

e Commence risperidone depot

8 A 25-year-old woman with a known history of cannabis misuse presents to A&E stating that David Beckham is madly in love with her and wants to marry her. What is the most likely diagnosis?

   a Capgras's syndrome

   b Cotard's syndrome

   c Erotomania

   d Fregoli's syndrome

   e Depression

9 The following are all factors associated with suicide EXCEPT:

   a An age greater than 40 years

   b Male gender

   c The winter season

   d Social class V

   e A recent life event such as divorce

10 The following are all factors associated with deliberate self-harm EXCEPT:

   a An age greater than 45 years

   b A recent life event such as divorce

   c Lower socioeconomic class

   d Unemployment

   e Female gender

11 A middle-aged gentleman presents to A&E following a recent overdose of 30 tablets of paracetamol. He states that he has been feeling low ever since he split up from his girlfriend. He comments that he has no reason to live and feels worthless. He is reviewed by the psychiatric doctor on call who admits him. He agrees to stay informally. While on the ward he becomes very restless and agitated and threatens to leave the hospital. With regard to the 1983 Mental Health Act what is the next most appropriate step in management?

a Section 136

b Section 2

c Section 3

d Section 5(2)

e Section 135

12 A patient with a known history of schizoaffective disorder is admitted to hospital following non-compliance with medication. Whilst on the ward the patient becomes verbally abusive to nursing staff and fellow patients. She states that she is not unwell and wants to leave. You advise the nursing staff that she requires sedative medication. She is given lorazepam and haloperidol intramuscularly as she is refusing it orally. Following such medication she is observed to have difficulty in initiating movement. What is the next most appropriate step in management?

a Baclofen

b Continue to observe

c Procyclidine

d Promethazine

e Diazepam

13 A 54-year-old woman presents to her GP complaining of poor sleep after losing her job. She comments that life is not worth living and that she sees no future. The patient is likely to demonstrate the following additional symptoms EXCEPT:

a Increased sexual promiscuity

b Weight loss

c Poor concentration

d Reduced energy

e Constipation

14 A middle-aged woman presents to her GP feeling low in mood. She has a background history of depression and has been prescribed citalopram 20 mg once daily. The following are all likely features of her mental state EXCEPT:

a Psychomotor retardation

b Delusional beliefs

c Auditory hallucinations

d Pressured speech

e Thoughts of self-harm

15 The following are all classical features of a major depressive episode EXCEPT:

a Weight gain

b Hypersomnia

c Reduced pleasure in day-to-day activities

d Suicidal ideation

e Feelings of worthlessness

16 The following are all factors associated with depression EXCEPT:

a A recent divorce

b An elderly age

c Female gender

d Limited social support

e A recent bereavement

17 A 35-year-old woman presents to her GP six weeks following childbirth. She complains of feeling low in mood and having poor sleep. On examination you note she is fairly unkempt in appearance, maintaining minimal eye contact and appears malnourished. Which management plan would you instigate first?

a Lithium

b ECT

c Cognitive behavioural therapy

d Venlafaxine

e Citalopram

18 A 45-year-old woman is admitted under Section 2 of the Mental Health Act following concerns raised by her husband. He states that she has been feeling low following a recent miscarriage and that she has made clear plans to end her life. She is prescribed citalopram 40 mg once daily. During the first week of her admission she is mute. She refuses oral medication and refuses to eat or drink. She appears notably dehydrated. The nursing staff report that she has not passed urine since admission and that her blood pressure is 95/70 mm Hg. Which management plan would you instigate first?

a Continue citalopram

b Commence olanzapine

c Cognitive behavioural therapy

d Psychosurgery

e ECT

19 A middle-aged woman is taken to A&E on a Section 136 following concerns raised by her boss at work. Whilst at work he noted that she was behaving bizarrely and was making comments of a sexual nature to fellow colleagues. At one point she removed all her clothes and began to do star jumps. She stated that she was the Queen of Egypt and could do as she pleased. The following are all likely features of her mental state examination EXCEPT:

a Psychomotor agitation

b Pressured speech

c Flight of ideas

d Psychomotor retardation

e Auditory hallucinations

20 A middle-aged woman is brought to A&E on a Section 136 following concerns about her behaviour. She was noted by her neighbours to be dancing in a ritualistic-like fashion on her balcony and throwing money and her belongings onto the street. Mental state assessment demonstrates evidence of an elated mood, pressured speech and psychomotor agitation. What is the most likely diagnosis?

a Depression

b Schizophrenia

c Bipolar affective disorder

d Personality disorder

e Delirium

21 A 45-year-old gentleman with a known history of bipolar affective disorder presents to his GP. On assessment the GP notes he is evidently thought disordered with pressured speech and psychomotor agitation. The patient states he has been non-compliant with his medication, namely lithium, for the past three months. What is the next most appropriate step in management?

a Fluoxetine

b Citalopram

c Olanzapine

d ECT

e Venlafaxine

22 A 23-year-old woman presents to her GP stating that she feels as if she has a foreign object within her stomach. She continues to state that she feels controlled by the object and that it tells her to harm others. Which management plan would you instigate first?

a Citalopram

b Lithium

c Clozapine

d Olanzapine

e Chlorpromazine

23 A middle-aged woman is taken to her GP by her mother following concerns of her mental state. During the consultation her mother states that her daughter has been mute while at home and on occasion grimaces and laughs inappropriately. During the consultation her daughter sits on the floor and begins to mutter incoherently. Which management plan would you instigate first?

a Amisulpride

b Clozapine

c Chlorpromazine

d Sodium valproate

e Haloperidol

24 A 25-year-old woman with a diagnosis of schizophrenia has been prescribed olanzapine 10 mg once at night. What is the most likely mode of action of olanzapine?

a Blockade of dopamine receptors

b Blockade of serotonin receptors

c Blockade of histamine receptors

d Blockade of acetylcholine receptors

e Blockade of prolactin receptors

25 A 54-year-old gentleman is referred to the mental health department by his GP following concerns in his mental state. He initially presented over four months ago stating that he is hearing voices telling him he is the King of Israel and that he has the ability to control people's thoughts. He was commenced initially on olanzapine for six weeks, which was then changed to quetiapine following no improvement in his mental state. During the consultation he continues to state he is the King of Israel and that he has been put on this earth to harm people. Which management plan would you instigate first?

a Continue quetiapine and review

b Commence risperidone

c Commence aripiprazole

d Commence clozapine

e Commence citalopram

26 The following are all common side-effects of antipsychotic drugs EXCEPT:

a Gynaecomastia

b Dry mouth

c Blurred vision

d Dystonia

e Diarrhoea

27 A newly diagnosed patient with schizophrenia presents to his GP complaining of a dry mouth and blurred vision. He has recently been commenced on olanzapine 10 mg at night. What is the most likely cause of his symptoms?

a Histamine blockade

b Dopamine blockade

c Serotonin blockade

d Acetylcholine blockade

e Prolactin blockade

28 A middle-aged gentleman with newly diagnosed schizophrenia presents to his GP complaining of reduced libido and breast enlargement. He has recently been commenced on risperidone 4 mg at night. What is the most likely cause of his symptoms?

a Histamine blockade

b Dopamine blockade

c Serotonin blockade

d Acetylcholine blockade

e Prolactin blockade

29 A middle-aged gentleman with a recent diagnosis of paranoid schizophrenia presents to his GP for a routine health check. During the consultation you note he is grimacing excessively with evidence of tongue protrusion and excessive eye blinking. Current medication includes olanzapine 10 mg at night. What is the most likely cause of his symptoms?

a Histamine blockade

b Dopamine blockade

c Serotonin blockade

d Acetylcholine blockade

e Prolactin blockade

30 You are a house officer on call in psychiatry when you are called by a nurse to review a patient urgently. She states that the patient is a known schizophrenic and is currently on risperidone 4 mg at night. She informs you that he has a temperature of 40° C. The patient is likely to demonstrate the following additional features EXCEPT:

a An altered conscious level

b Bradycardia

c Muscular rigidity

d Urinary incontinence

e Pallor

31 You are a senior house officer on call in medicine when you are referred a patient from the psychiatric ward. The patient has a background history of paranoid schizophrenia and is on olanzapine. He currently has a temperature of 38° C and has a fluctuating conscious level. The following are all likely to be common blood abnormalities EXCEPT:

a A raised white cell count

b Deranged liver function

c A raised creatine phosphokinase level

d A raised haemoglobin level

e A raised neutrophil count

32 A 34-year-old woman is admitted to the mental health ward. She has a past history of schizophrenia and has been trialled on risperidone and more recently quetiapine over the past few months. She appears notably thought disordered. The consultant decides to commence clozapine. What is the next most appropriate initial investigation prior to starting clozapine?

a Electrocardiogram

b Chest X-ray

c Echocardiogram

d Thyroid function tests

e Liver function tests

33 A patient has been recently commenced on clozapine. The pharmacist asks you to monitor the patient's bloods while on clozapine. What is the next most appropriate initial blood investigation?

a Thyroid function tests

b Serum ferritin

c Full blood count

d Hepatitis screen

e Liver function tests

34 A 55-year-old woman presents to A&E stating that she can see a dark figure in her home. She states the figure talks to her and stands next to her bed. She continues to say the figure makes her fearful and has been threatening to harm her. She has a past medical history of ischaemic heart disease, hypertension and dementia. What is the next most appropriate step in management?

a Risperidone

b Olanzapine

c Amisulpride

d Quetiapine

e Haloperidol

35 The following are all common side-effects of atypical antipsychotics EXCEPT:

a Weight loss

b Hyperglycaemia

c Sedation

d Dry mouth

e Constipation

36 A 35-year-old woman presents to A&E following non-compliance with her lithium. Mental state examination reveals that she is notably thought disordered, pressured in speech with evidence of psychomotor agitation. You decide to restart her lithium. The following are all important to monitor with regard to lithium EXCEPT:

a Serum urea

b Thyroid function tests

c Lithium levels

d Liver function tests

e Serum creatinine

37 The following are all common side-effects of lithium EXCEPT:

a Dry mouth

b Polyuria

c Polydypsia

d Weight loss

e Oedema

38 A middle-aged woman with a known history of mental illness presents to A&E complaining of a metallic taste in her mouth. She also states that she has been feeling particularly nauseous recently. She comments that she is on medication for her mental illness but she cannot remember the name of the tablet. What is the most likely drug responsible for her symptoms?

a Olanzapine

b Risperidone

c Lithium ✓

d Quetiapine

e Sodium valproate

39 You are a house officer in psychiatry when you admit a patient with a history of bipolar affective disorder. She has re-presented following non-compliance with medication and subsequent deterioration in her mental state. Normal medication includes lithium 600 mg at night. You discuss the case with the registrar on call who asks you to recommence the lithium and then perform a lithium level. When should a lithium level be most ideally performed?

a 1 hour post-dose

b 2 hours post-dose

c 4 hours post-dose

d 6 hours post-dose

e 8 hours post-dose ✓ 8 - 12 hrs

40 A patient with a known history of bipolar affective disorder takes lithium 800 mg at night. What is the most appropriate therapeutic plasma range of lithium?

a 0.1–0.2 mmol/L

b 0.2–0.4 mmol/L

c 0.4–1.0 mmol/L

d 1–2 mmol/L

e 2–3 mmol/L

41 The following are all signs of lithium toxicity EXCEPT:

a Tinnitus

b Blurred vision

c Constipation

d Tremor

e Muscle weakness

42 A patient with a known history of bipolar affective disorder is commenced on carbamazepine in combination with lithium. The following are all important with regard to carbamazepine blood monitoring EXCEPT:

a Liver function tests

b White cell count

c Platelet count

d Haemoglobin levels

e Vitamin D levels

43 A middle-aged woman with a known history of bipolar affective disorder re-presents to her GP complaining of visual disturbances. On examination you note redness of her conjunctiva bilaterally. She has recently been commenced on a new medication for her mental illness. What is the most likely drug responsible for her symptoms?

a   Olanzapine

b   Carbamazapine

c   Lithium

d   Sodium valproate

e   Citalopram

44 What is the most likely mode of action of tricyclic antidepressant medication?

a   Inhibition of serotonin reuptake alone

b   Inhibition of noradrenaline reuptake alone

c   Inhibition of histamine reuptake alone

d   Inhibition of serotonin and noradrenaline reuptake

e   Inhibition of dopamine reuptake

45 A 45-year-old gentleman presents to his GP. He has recently lost his job and has been evicted from his accommodation. He has a known history of depression and is currently on citalopram 20 mg daily. He states he feels so low that he wants to end his life and has contemplated taking an overdose of paracetamol. However, he states that he would not act on such intention because of his love for his wife. You decide to change his medication and commence him on imipramine. You inform him he needs an electrocardiogram (ECG) to ensure no cardiovascular side-effects of the medication. What is the most likely cardiovascular abnormality that may be noted on the ECG?

   a T wave flattening

   b Peaked P waves

   c ST elevation

   d Absent P waves

   e Q waves

46 A 42-year-old woman with a background history of depression presents to her GP complaining of a black tongue and nausea. She has been recently started on a new antidepressant medication. What is the most likely drug responsible for her symptoms?

   a Venlafaxine

   b Imipramine

   c Citalopram

   d Fluoxetine

   e Reboxetine

47 Which one of the following drugs is an example of a selective noradrenaline and serotonin reuptake inhibitor?

a Venlafaxine

b Imipramine

c Citalopram

d Fluoxetine

e Reboxetine

48 A newly diagnosed depressive patient is referred to the out-patient department for routine blood tests. Investigations reveal a platelet count of 100×10^9/L. He has been recently started on new medication for his depression. What is the most likely drug responsible for such blood results?

a Venlafaxine

b Reboxetine

c Mirtazapine

d Imipramine

e Fluoxetine

49 A 32-year-old gentleman presents to his GP feeling generally unwell. He has a background history of depression and has been recently started on a new medication for his depression. Routine observations reveal a pulse rate of 87 beats per minute and blood pressure of 190/80 mm Hg. He comments he has been drinking heavily recently to help lift his spirits. What is the most likely drug responsible for such findings?

a Phenelzine

b Reboxetine

c Mirtazapine

d Imipramine

e Fluoxetine

50 You are the house officer on call in medicine when you are asked to clerk a patient who has been referred by his GP following an abnormal blood pressure reading. On examination you note a blood pressure of 195/85 mm Hg. He has a past medical history of depression, hayfever and eczema. He comments he has been using a nasal decongestant spray recently to help alleviate his hayfever symptoms. You question him with regard to current medication for his depression, which he is unable to recall. What is the most likely drug responsible for such a presentation?

a Phenelzine

b Reboxetine

c Mirtazapine

d Imipramine

e Fluoxetine

51 A patient with a known history of depression has been recently commenced on phenelzine. On examination you note his blood pressure is 195/110 mm Hg. He has a history of chronic alcohol misuse. What is the next most appropriate step in management?

    a Commence a beta blocker

    b Commence an ACE inhibitor

    c Stop phenelzine and commence olanzapine

    d Stop phenelzine and commence moclobemide

    e Monitor blood pressure and review in a week

52 Which of the following is an example of a short-acting benzodiazepine?

    a Diazepam

    b Chlordiazepoxide

    c Lorazepam

    d Nitrazepam

    e Olanzapine

53 Which one of the following neurotransmitters is involved in the mode of action of diazepam?

    a Acetylcholine

    b Dopamine

    c GABA

    d Histamine

    e Serotonin

54 A 35-year-old woman presents to A&E complaining of low mood, appetite loss and tinnitus. She comments that she does not feel real and that the surrounding environment is not real. She has a history of mental illness. She states that for the past month she has stopped taking her medication but she cannot recall the name of the drug. What is the most likely drug responsible for such a presentation?

a Olanzapine

b Risperidone

c Lithium

d Diazepam

e Quetiapine

55 The following are all common side-effects of ECT EXCEPT:

a Headache

b Confusion

c Memory loss

d Nausea

e Weight loss

56 The following are all contraindications of ECT EXCEPT:

a Recent myocardial infarction

b Cerebral aneurysm

c Chest infection

d Cardiac arrhythmias

e Hypothyroidism

57 A middle-aged woman with a working diagnosis of depression presents to the outpatient psychiatric department stating that she feels low in mood with poor appetite and minimal energy. She has been taking venlafaxine 37.5 mg twice daily for the past six months. She feels the medication is of no use and would like to be referred for cognitive behavioural therapy. She states she feels guilty ever since she cheated on her husband. What is the most likely term used to describe this presentation?

a Arbitrary interference

b Personalisation

c Selective abstraction

d Maximisation

e Catastrophising

58 A 35-year-old woman is referred to the psychiatric ward by her GP following concerns in her mental state. She is currently 35 weeks pregnant. During the consultation she states that she wants to harm the baby and that when she watches television she sees messages on the screen telling her to act on such thoughts. She is admitted under Section 2 of the Mental Health Act. Which management plan would you instigate first?

a Risperidone

b Olanzapine

c Quetiapine

d Citalopram

e Aripiprazole

59 A 25-year-old woman presents to her GP complaining of feeling
low in mood and worthless. She has recently given birth to her
first child. The GP is concerned about the possibility of postnatal depression (PND). What is the most likely timeframe for
the occurrence of PND?

a 1–2 weeks post-partum

b 10–12 weeks post-partum

c 14–16 weeks post-partum

d 2–6 weeks post-partum

e 6–8 hours post-partum

60 A 16-year-old girl is brought to her GP by her mother following concerns about her weight. During the consultation the girl
comments she is fearful of becoming overweight and has been
exercising for five hours per day. You are concerned about the
possibility of anorexia nervosa. What is the following ICD-10
criterion for body weight with regard to anorexia nervosa?

a 5% below expected weight

b 10% below expected weight

c 15% below expected weight

d 20% below expected weight

e 25% below expected weight

61 The following are all common gastrointestinal complications of anorexia nervosa EXCEPT:

a Diarrhoea

b Gastric dilatation

c Delayed gastric emptying

d Delayed small bowel transit time

e Acute pancreatitis

62 An 18-year-old girl is admitted to the mental health ward following concerns about her weight. She admits to using laxatives to help her lose weight and purging as she feels obese. On examination you note she is severely emaciated with evidence of lanugo hair on her face. You perform routine blood investigations. What is the most likely abnormality noted from blood investigation?

a Thrombocytosis

b Hypocholesterolaemia

c Hypokalaemia

d Hypermagnesaemia

e Low albumin

63 A patient with newly diagnosed anorexia nervosa complains of feeling dizzy. Routine observations reveal a pulse rate of 110 beats per minute and a blood pressure of 85/45 mm Hg. You decide to perform an ECG. The following abnormalities are most likely to be noted on the ECG EXCEPT:

a ST elevation

b T wave flattening

c T wave inversion

d Prolonged QT interval

e QT slope enhancement

64 A 19-year-old woman presents to her GP stating that she feels fat. She admits to overeating and then purging. On examination you note evidence of calluses on the dorsum of her right hand. What is the term most likely used to describe such a finding?

a Grey Turner's sign

b Cullen's sign

c Russell's sign

d Murphy's sign

e Rovsing's sign

65 An 18-year-old girl presents to her GP with preoccupations about her weight. She states that she feels overweight and wants to end her life. During the consultation she admits to using laxatives and on occasion binge eating. On examination you note evidence of salivary gland swelling and poor dental hygiene. Which management plan would you instigate first?

a Citalopram 20 mg once daily

b Fluoxetine 60 mg once daily

c Olanzapine 10 mg once daily

d Risperidone 4 mg once daily

e Lithium 800 mg once daily

66 A 25-year-old gentleman presents to A&E stating that he can see a shadow of his ex-girlfriend while he sleeps. He continues to say that the shadow moves particular objects around his flat and commands him to steal. You end the consultation and attempt to shake the patient's hand. You observe that he extends his hand as if to shake yours but then withdraws. He continues to perform this action repeatedly. What is the term most appropriately used to describe such an action?

a Echopraxia

b Ambitendency

c Posturing

d Waxy flexibility

e Mannerism

67 A patient with a recent diagnosis of schizophrenia is admitted to hospital under Section 3 of the Mental Health Act following non-compliance with medication. You perform a general physical health check as part of his formal clerking and note that during assessment of his power his body feels like soft wax and then stiffens. What is the term most appropriately used to describe such a finding?

a Echopraxia

b Ambitendency

c Posturing

d Waxy flexibility

e Mannerism

68 A middle-aged life-long alcoholic presents to A&E following a drinking binge. He is commenced on a detox regime and formally admitted. Two days later he appears notably agitated and states he feels deafened by the general noise on the ward. He also comments the lights on the ward are too bright and that he can see strange shapes on the wall. What is the most likely diagnosis?

a Schizophrenia

b Depression

c Bipolar affective disorder

d Dementia

e Delirium

69 The following are all common metabolic causes of delirium EXCEPT:

a Hepatic failure

b Vitamin D deficiency

c Vitamin B12 deficiency

d Cardiac failure

e Renal failure

70 A 70-year-old gentleman is brought to A&E by his carer following concerns in his behaviour. During your assessment you note he is unable to tell you the time or tell you where he is. He comments that he feels the doctors and nurses are all against him and want to kill him. What is the most likely diagnosis?

a Schizophrenia

b Dementia

c Hypothyroidism

d Bipolar affective disorder

e Depression

71 A 65-year-old woman presents to A&E following concerns by her GP. During the consultation you note she is disorientated in time, place and person. She is unable to recall her date of birth or where she lives. She also comments that she feels the Prime Minister Gordon Brown wants to kill her for refusing to use public transport. You are concerned about the possibility of dementia. What is the most likely type of dementia she is suffering from?

a Diffuse Lewy body dementia

b Alzheimer's disease

c Vascular dementia

d Frontotemporal dementia

e Parietal dementia

72 With regard to Alzheimer's disease what is the most likely pathological finding?

a Accumulation of delta amyloid protein

b Accumulation of omega amyloid protein

c Accumulation of delta and beta amyloid protein

d Accumulation of alpha amyloid protein

e Accumulation of beta amyloid protein

73 A 75-year-old gentleman is reviewed by his GP for a routine blood pressure check. During the consultation you note that he appears confused and disorientated. He is unable to recall his name or address. You also observe that he has difficulty in naming simple objects such as your pen and your watch. What is the next most appropriate step in management?

a Donepezil

b Risperidone

c Continue to observe

d Quetiapine

e Urine drug screen

74 A 72-year-old woman is recently diagnosed with Alzheimer's disease. You decide to commence her on memantine. What is the most likely mechanism of action of memantine?

a Dopamine antagonist

b Serotonin antagonist

c Acetylcholine antagonist

d NMDA antagonist

e Histamine antagonist

75 A 71-year-old woman is recently diagnosed with Alzheimer's disease. You decide to commence her on rivastigmine. What is the most likely mechanism of action of rivastigmine?

a Dopamine antagonist

b NMDA antagonist

c Acetylcholine antagonist

d Histamine antagonist

e Acetylcholinesterase inhibitor

76 A 67-year-old gentleman presents to his GP complaining of seeing spiders every time he goes to bed. On examination you note evidence of an expressionless face. What is the most likely diagnosis?

a Alzheimer's disease

b Frontotemporal dementia

c Vascular dementia

d Schizophrenia

e Lewy body dementia

77 A 65-year-old gentleman is brought to his GP following concerns raised by his wife. She comments that he seems like a different person. She states that he does not seem to pay attention to her anymore and is often quite withdrawn. During the consultation you note he is essentially mute with poverty of movement. What is the most likely diagnosis?

   a Alzheimer's disease

   b Frontotemporal dementia

   c Vascular dementia

   d Schizophrenia

   e Lewy body dementia

78 A 75-year-old woman is seen by her GP following concerns raised by her carer. The carer states that she appears notably confused and disorientated in time and place. She has a past medical history of hypertension and ischaemic heart disease. What is the most likely diagnosis?

   a Alzheimer's disease

   b Frontotemporal dementia

   c Vascular dementia

   d Schizophrenia

   e Lewy body dementia

79 A chronic alcohol abuser presents to his GP for a routine check up. During the consultation you ask him how things have been generally and he is unable to comment. He states he can barely remember what day it is. You ask him to repeat the following address, '12A Berkeley Square House, Berkeley Square, London', and repeat it five minutes later. He is able to do so. What is the most likely diagnosis?

a Wernicke's encephalopathy

b Frontotemporal dementia

c Schizophrenia

d Korsakov's syndrome

e Lewy body dementia

80 With regard to the above question what is the most likely aetiological cause of his symptoms?

a Vitamin D deficiency

b Vitamin A deficiency

c Vitamin E deficiency

d Vitamin K deficiency

e Vitamin B1 deficiency

81 An elderly woman presents to A&E following concerns by her carer. She appears elated in mood but irritable. She seems to be involved in some form of verbal altercation with her carer, which is abusive in nature. During the consultation you note that she repeats her name with increased frequency. What is the most likely aetiological cause for this presentation?

a Frontal lobe damage

b Temporal lobe damage

c Occipital lobe damage

d Parietal lobe damage

e Subarachnoid haemorrhage

82 An elderly gentleman presents to his GP complaining that he is no longer able to read properly. He states that he can see words but has difficulty reading them. During the consultation you observe that he speaks fluently but is unable to understand questions you ask him. What is the most likely aetiological cause for this presentation?

a Frontal lobe damage

b Temporal lobe damage

c Occipital lobe damage

d Parietal lobe damage

e Subarachnoid haemorrhage

83 An elderly gentleman presents to his GP following concerns raised by his carer. She comments that he has lost his ability to write even though he can read well. Routine examination demonstrates evidence of finger agnosia and right-to-left disorientation. What additional feature is he most likely to demonstrate?

a Sensory aphasia

b Metamorphopsia

c Urinary incontinence

d Dyscalculia

e Hypersomnia

84 What is the most likely aetiological cause for the above presentation?

a Frontal lobe damage

b Temporal lobe damage

c Occipital lobe damage

d Parietal lobe damage

e Subarachnoid haemorrhage

85 An elderly gentleman is brought to A&E by his wife following concerns about a change in his behaviour. He states that he can see flames and the devil in the evening. He also points at your tie and asks if it is a knife. What additional feature is he most likely to demonstrate?

a Auditory hallucinations

b Prosopagnosia

c Urinary incontinence

d Dyscalculia

e Hypersomnia

86 What is the most likely aetiological cause for the above presentation?

    a Frontal lobe damage

    b Temporal lobe damage

    c Occipital lobe damage

    d Parietal lobe damage

    e Subarachnoid haemorrhage

87 An elderly patient presents complaining of increased pain and discomfort whenever he goes to pick up the kettle or butter his toast. He states this has never happened to him before and he is concerned about what it could be. You inform him that it is commonly known as hyperalgesia. What is the most likely aetiological cause for his symptoms?

    a Frontal lobe damage

    b Temporal lobe damage

    c Occipital lobe damage

    d Parietal lobe damage

    e Thalamic damage

88 A 32-year-old woman presents to A&E complaining that she is being followed by members of Arsenal football team and that she has been sexually assaulted by three of the footballers so far. She has a history of long-standing cannabis misuse. You are concerned about the possibility of acute psychosis and decide to section her. What is the most appropriate section of the Mental Health Act in this case?

a Section 2

b Section 3

c Section 4

d Section 5(2)

e Section 136

89 What is the maximum length of time patients can be held under Section 2 of the Mental Health Act?

a 7 days

b 10 days

c 20 days

d 24 days

e 28 days

90 Which of the following statements most closely applies to Section 2 of the Mental Health Act?

a A section for treatment

b A section for assessment

c A section to enable individuals to be removed from a public place to a place of safety for assessment

d A holding section if a patient threatens to leave hospital

e A section for emergency admission

91 A 32-year-old woman is brought to A&E by her partner following concerns about her behaviour in the past few weeks. He comments that she has been stripping inappropriately in public places. Her mother has a history of bipolar affective disorder. You admit her informally to the mental health ward. She threatens to leave and so you place her under a Section 5(2). After 72 hours the section has lapsed and she continues to state that she wants to leave and will commit suicide on the ward if she is not discharged. You make a recommendation for a Section 2. Which of the following people are required for a Section 2 recommendation?

a Nearest relative

b One medical practitioner

c Two medical practitioners

d Police officer

e Patient's former school head teacher

92 A patient has been placed under Section 2 of the Mental Health Act. You explain that she has every right to appeal her section. What is the most likely time frame for appeal?

a Within 2 days

b Within 4 days

c Within 6 days

d Within 10 days

e Within 14 days

93 A middle-aged woman has been found running in and out of traffic screaming incoherently. You are a passer by and call the police. The police inform you that they will take her to hospital under a section of the Mental Health Act. What is the most appropriate section of the Mental Health Act that should be used?

a Section 2

b Section 3

c Section 4

d Section 136

e Section 135

94 A chronic schizophrenic is placed under a section of the Mental Health Act following concerns in her mental state. She comments that the BBC has cameras that are keeping her under surveillance and watch her while she sleeps. Her care coordinator informs you that she has been non-compliant with her depot medication risperidone. What is the most likely section of the Mental Health Act that the patient has been placed under?

a Section 2

b Section 3

c Section 4

d Section 5(2)

e Section 136

95 With regard to the above section, what is the most likely time-frame that it lasts for?

a 1 month

b 2 months

c 4 months

d 5 months

e 6 months

96 A patient has been placed under Section 3 of the Mental Health Act following lapse of her Section 2. Who is most likely able to appeal such a decision?

a The patient's neighbour

b The patient's work boss

c The patient's nearest relative

d The patient's school headteacher

e The patient's hairdresser

97 You are the house officer on call in psychiatry and have been called by your registrar. He informs you that he has admitted a patient from clinic under section as an emergency admission for assessment. What is the most likely section of the Mental Health Act that has been used?

a Section 2

b Section 3

c Section 4

d Section 5(2)

e Section 136

98 With regard to the above named section, what is the most likely timeframe that it can last for?

a 1 month

b 2 weeks

c 48 hours

d 24 hours

e 72 hours

99 A middle-aged woman presents to her GP complaining of feeling fearful when she leaves her home. She states that she feels uncomfortable in crowds and public places. What is the most likely diagnosis?

a Agoraphobia

b Social phobia

c Specific phobia

d Panic disorder

e Generalised anxiety disorder

100 A 20-year-old woman presents to her GP stating that she feels fearful when she enters shops or travels on public transport. She comments that she feels well within herself, is sleeping and eating well and has no thoughts of self-harm or suicidal intent. What is the next most appropriate step in management?

a Olanzapine

b Diazepam

c Citalopram

d Fluoxetine

e Behavioural therapy

101 A 30-year-old woman presents to her GP. She has recently started a new job as a primary care policy advisor for the Department of Health. She comments that she dislikes her job as it involves chairing meetings and speaking in conferences at a local and national level. She states that she thinks people are also criticising her although she admits that no one has directly said anything of the sort. What is the most likely diagnosis?

a Agoraphobia

b Social phobia

c Specific phobia

d Panic disorder

e Generalised anxiety disorder

102 What is the next most appropriate step in management for the above patient?

a Olanzapine

b Diazepam

c Citalopram

d Fluoxetine

e Behavioural therapy

103 A 30-year-old woman presents to her GP stating that she has recently been suffering from episodes of palpitations, shortness of breath and sweating. She comments that these episodes last for a few minutes but she feels like she is going to die. She has no known past medical history. What is the most likely diagnosis?

   a Agoraphobia

   b Social phobia

   c Specific phobia

   d Panic disorder

   e Generalised anxiety disorder

104 A 32-year-old gentleman presents to his GP complaining of long-standing episodes of palpitations, chest pain and dizziness. He has no known past medical history. He is a non-smoker and non-drinker. He has recently changed his GP as he felt that his previous GP did not take his symptoms seriously. He states he is feeling otherwise well, maintains a good appetite and is sleeping well. What is the next most appropriate step in management?

   a Olanzapine

   b Lithium

   c Diazepam

   d Imipramine

   e Propranolol

105 A 30-year-old woman has recently been diagnosed with generalised anxiety disorder. The following are all features of generalised anxiety disorder EXCEPT:

a Dry mouth

b Constipation

c Urinary frequency

d Shortness of breath

e Dizziness

106 A 32-year-old woman presents to her GP. She has a long-standing history of palpitations, dizziness and shortness of breath. She is unable to ascertain a trigger for such symptoms. During the consultation she complains of feeling sweaty and experiencing abdominal discomfort. Routine observations reveal a blood pressure of 125/75 mm Hg and a pulse rate of 125 beats per minute. She has been trialled on diazepam and imipramine in the past. What is the next most appropriate step in management?

a Propranolol alone

b Olanzapine

c Continue imipramine

d Propranolol and refer for cognitive behavioural therapy

e Lithium

107 A 32-year-old woman presents to her GP following concerns raised by her husband. He states that she spends most of her day pre-occupied with cleaning the house. She feels that there are germs everywhere and washes her hands up to eight times a day. On examination you note evidence of erythema and excoriation of both her palms. What is the most likely diagnosis?

a Schizophrenia

b Depression

c Generalised anxiety disorder

d Obsessive compulsive disorder

e Acute stress reaction

108 Which management plan would you instigate first in the above patient?

a Psychosurgery

b Citalopram

c Olanzapine

d Sodium valproate

e Venlafaxine

109 A 45-year-old Turkish gentleman presents to the psychiatric outpatient department. He comments that he feels low in mood and experiences palpitations on occasion. He states that this has been long-lasting and came on after he was taken prisoner in Turkey and tortured. As a result of this experience he fled to the UK to seek asylum. He comments that whenever he sleeps he experiences flashbacks of the event. What is the most likely diagnosis?

a Obsessive compulsive disorder

b Panic disorder

c Acute stress reaction

d Post traumatic stress reaction

e Generalised anxiety disorder

110 A middle-aged woman presents to her GP. She complains of feeling low in mood and having poor sleep. She also comments that she experiences episodes of palpitations and shortness of breath. She has recently lost her husband and states that her symptoms have occurred ever since his passing. What is the most likely diagnosis?

a Conversion disorder

b Adjustment disorder

c Acute stress reaction

d Post-traumatic stress reaction

e Generalised anxiety disorder

111 A 54-year-old gentleman is brought to his GP by his wife following concerns in his behaviour. She comments that he has been seeing shadows of his father, who passed away several years ago, each afternoon and states that he has been communicating with these shadows on occasion. You assess his cognitive function and note that when you ask him how many numbers a clock face has, he replies 14. You then ask him how many months there are in a calendar year and he replies 17. However, you note that he is orientated in time, place and person. What is the most likely diagnosis?

a Multiple personality disorder

b Ganser's syndrome

c Dissociative amnesia

d Subdural haematoma

e Schizophrenia

112 A 26-year-old woman presents to her GP. She is a new patient to the practice but from her records you note she has no known past medical or surgical history. She is on no current medication and has no known drug allergies. She is very distressed and states that she is having a heart attack. She also complains of stomach pain and thinks she is dying of stomach and bowel cancer. What is the most likely diagnosis?

a Somatization disorder

b Hypochondrial disorder

c Persistent somatoform pain disorder

d Acute psychosis

e Depression

113 A specialist registrar in medicine presents to his GP. He states he feels low in mood as he has not been shortlisted as a consultant at the Hammersmith Hospital in London. He comments that he was treated unfairly during the interview. He also states that he feels his wife has been cheating on him recently as he has been focusing on his work too much and neglecting the relationship. However, he is not able to confirm this as true. What is the most likely diagnosis?

a   Schizoid personality disorder

b   Paranoid personality disorder

c   Dissocial personality disorder

d   Histrionic personality disorder

e   Emotionally unstable personality disorder

114 A 25-year-old gentleman presents to his GP feeling tearful and low in mood. He has recently moved to London and states it is the best city in the world. However, he comments that he finds people boring and antisocial. He continues by saying people rarely want to spend their money and refuse to go to Michelin-starred restaurants and expensive bars. During the consultation, he continually interrupts you to talk about himself and to check his appearance in the mirror. What is the most likely diagnosis?

a   Schizoid personality disorder

b   Paranoid personality disorder

c   Dissocial personality disorder

d   Histrionic personality disorder

e   Emotionally unstable personality disorder

115 A fifth-year medical student presents to her GP feeling low in mood. She has recently split up from her boyfriend who is currently a foundation year one doctor. She comments that she feels really stressed at the moment as she is due to apply for jobs and hand in her coursework assignments. She states that she used to rely on her boyfriend for everything and now that he has gone she won't be able to do such things by herself. What is the most likely diagnosis?

a Schizoid personality disorder

b Dependent personality disorder

c Dissocial personality disorder

d Histrionic personality disorder

e Emotionally unstable personality disorder

116 A chronic alcohol abuser presents to A&E complaining of epigastric pain following an alcoholic binge. You place him on a detox regime of chlordiazepoxide and pabrinex. Two days later he is notably tremulous and complains of worsened abdominal discomfort and nausea. What term most appropriately describes this presentation?

a Tolerance

b Withdrawal

c Dependence

d Intoxication

e Psychosis

117 A 35-year-old Polish builder presents to A&E following an alcoholic binge. He comments he loves alcohol and it keeps him going in life. What term most appropriately describes this presentation?

a Tolerance

b Withdrawal

c Dependence

d Intoxication

e Psychosis

118 A 25-year-old crack cocaine user presents to his GP stating that he needs a letter to apply for income support. He has recently lost his job at Goldman Sachs following drug misuse at work and is unable to find further employment. He comments that he has been spending more money on his drug habit and using a larger amount to get the same rush. What term most appropriately describes this presentation?

a Tolerance

b Withdrawal

c Dependence

d Intoxication

e Psychosis

119 A chronic alcohol misuser presents to A&E following a drinking binge. Routine blood investigations reveal a haemoglobin of 10 g/dL. What is the most likely additional blood abnormality?

    a Low mean corpuscular volume

    b Neutrophilia

    c Thrombocytosis

    d Low serum folate

    e Raised serum calcium

120 The following are all features of Wernicke's encephalopathy EXCEPT:

    a Nystagmus

    b Ataxia

    c Exopthalmus

    d Opthalmoplegia

    e Peripheral neuropathy

121 The following are all features of alcohol dependency EXCEPT:

    a Increased tolerance to alcohol

    b Repeated withdrawal symptoms

    c Reinstatement of drinking after abstinence

    d Primacy of drinking over other activities

    e A widening of the drinking repertoire

122 The following psychiatric disorders are all predisposing factors towards alcohol dependency EXCEPT:

a Depression

b Anxiety

c Schizophrenia

d Hypermania

e Phobia

123 A chronic alcohol misuser presents to his GP requesting treatment for his addiction. You discuss the possibility of psychotherapy or medical therapy with disulfiram. You inform him that if he continues to drink alcohol while taking disulfiram he will experience some unpleasant side-effects. The following are all likely side-effects EXCEPT:

a Bradycardia

b Headache

c Nausea

d Vomiting

e Facial flushing

124 A chronic alcohol misuser presents to his GP requesting disulfiram. You explain that while taking such medication he must abstain from alcohol otherwise he will experience unpleasant side-effects. He agrees to abstain. One week later he re-presents and says that he experienced a headache and severe vomiting with the medication. He admits to drinking alcohol during this time. What is the most likely aetiological cause for his symptoms?

a Serotonin release

b Acetaldehyde accumulation

c Noradrenaline blockade

d Histamine release

e Dopamine blockade

125 A 25-year-old woman is rushed to A&E following a sudden collapse. On examination you note small pinpoint pupils and evidence of needle marks on both arms and legs. What is the most likely diagnosis?

a Heroin overdose

b Paracetamol overdose

c Diazepam overdose

d Alcohol intoxication

e Cocaine overdose

126 A middle-aged woman presents to her GP stating that she is being followed by members of the Beatles pop group. During the consultation she repeatedly asks you for food stating that she could eat for England. What is the most likely diagnosis?

a Heroin misuse

b Cocaine overdose

c Diazepam overdose

d Alcohol intoxication

e Cannabis misuse

127 A 26-year-old city worker presents to A&E complaining of central crushing chest pain. Chest examination reveals normal heart sounds with no tenderness on chest wall palpation. An ECG demonstrates normal sinus rhythm. A troponin taken 12 hours post-onset is 0.09 µg/L. What is the most likely aetiological cause?

a Cocaine misuse

b Diazepam overdose

c Alcohol intoxication

d Cannabis misuse

e None of the above

128 A 21-year-old man presents to A&E. He has recently been to an underground rave event. On examination you note evidence of dilated pupils. Routine observations reveal a blood pressure of 125/65 mm Hg and pulse rate of 110 beats per minute. During the consultation he asks you whether the doctors and nurses are real. What is the most likely aetiological cause for this presentation?

a Cocaine misuse

b MDMA misuse

c Alcohol intoxication

d Cannabis misuse

e Diazepam overdose

129 The following are all features of pseudodementia EXCEPT:

a Low mood

b Rapid progression of symptoms

c Evidence of cerebral atrophy

d Memory loss

e Distress conveyance

130 The following are all features of Alzheimer's disease EXCEPT:

a Labile mood

b Ventricular enlargement

c Memory loss

d A normal electroencephalogram (EEG)

e Slow progression of symptoms

131 A 10-year-old child is brought to his GP following concerns raised by his school teacher. His teacher has commented that he runs around the class, barely listens to instructions and is easily distracted by other classmates. What is the most likely diagnosis?

    a Attention deficit hyperactivity disorder

    b Pica

    c Conduct disorder

    d Bipolar affective disorder

    e None of the above

132 A nine-year-old girl is brought to her GP following concerns raised by her school teacher. Her teacher comments that she is very threatening to other classmates and often starts physical fights. There has also been one incident whereby she has set fire to books in the school library. What is the most likely diagnosis?

    a Attention deficit hyperactivity disorder

    b Pica

    c Conduct disorder

    d Bipolar affective disorder

    e None of the above

133 A 10-year-old boy is recently diagnosed with conduct disorder. Which management plan would you instigate first?

a Lithium

b Olanzapine

c Methylphenidate

d Dexamfetamine

e Psychotherapy

134 A six-year-old boy is brought to the GP by his mother. She comments that he has wet the bed at least twice a week for the past three months. He is otherwise well and maintains a good appetite and sleeps well. A urine dipstick reveals no evidence of infection. What is the most likely aetiological cause for his symptoms?

a Abnormal bladder weakness

b Genetic factors

c Depression

d Abnormal bladder size

e Insufficient toilet training by mother

135 A 10-year-old girl is recently diagnosed with functional enuresis. Which management plan would you instigate first?

a A tricyclic antidepressant

b A selective serotonin reuptake inhibitor

c An antipsychotic

d A diuretic

e Paracetamol

136 A middle-aged gentleman with a background history of schizophrenia is seen in the outpatient department. During the consultation you note he mimics the exact same movement you carry out. What term most appropriately describes such a behaviour?

a Ambitendency

b Echopraxia

c Mannerism

d Negativism

e Posturing

137 You are the psychiatric house officer on call when you are asked to review a patient. Mental state examination reveals a well dressed, kempt female with good eye contact and rapport. You note her speech is fluent but rambling in nature. What term most appropriately describes such a phenomenon?

a Pressure of speech

b Logorrhoea

c Dysprosody

d Poverty of speech

e Dysarthria

138 A 23-year-old Afro-Caribbean woman presents to A&E. She states that she lives on the streets to help her become 'pubertated' and states that her mother is white and her father is black which makes her 'caucasic'. What term most appropriately describes such a presentation?

a Passing by the point

b Talking past the point

c Dysarthria

d Neologism

e Palilalia

139 A 32-year-old cannabis misuser presents stating that her arms can control the Queen of England and that she uses her hands to communicate with the BBC. What term most appropriately describes such a phenomenon?

a Delusion of poverty

b Delusion of reference

c Somatic delusion

d Delusion of grandeur

e Delusion of doubles

140 A middle-aged woman presents stating that her thoughts are being controlled by the FBI and that she feels they are taking part in her thinking process. What term most appropriately describes such a phenomenon?

a Thought alienation

b Made feelings

c Made impulses

d Made actions

e Somatic passivity

141 A middle-aged gentleman presents stating that he believes to be greater than Prince Charles and has been asked by God Himself to rule the world. What term most appropriately describes such a phenomenon?

a Delusion of poverty

b Delusion of reference

c Somatic delusion

d Delusion of grandeur

e Delusion of doubles

142 A patient with known schizophrenia presents to his GP. During the consultation you note his speech is an odd mixture of words and phrases. What term most appropriately describes such a phenomenon?

a Knight's move thinking

b Word salad

c Pressured speech

d Echolalia

e Thought blocking

143 A 24-year-old man with a background history of schizophrenia attends a routine outpatient follow-up appointment. During the consultation you note the patient stops suddenly midway through conversation and fails to recall what was being discussed. What term most appropriately describes such a phenomenon?

a Knight's move thinking

b Word salad

c Pressured speech

d Echolalia

e Thought blocking

144 A schizophrenic patient presents to his GP. During the consultation you note evidence of thought disorder with no true connection between the patient's thoughts and ideas. What term most appropriately describes such a phenomenon?

a Knight's move thinking

b Word salad

c Pressured speech

d Echolalia

e Thought blocking

145 A 32-year-old woman with a history of bipolar affective disorder presents to her GP following non-compliance with medication. During the consultation you note her speech is extremely rapid in nature and that she converses about several different topics. What term most appropriately describes such a phenomenon?

a Knight's move thinking

b Word salad

c Flight of ideas

d Pressured speech

e Thought blocking

146 A patient with a known history of mental illness presents to his GP. During the consultation you note he imitates your speech exactly. What term most appropriately describes such a phenomenon?

a Knight's move thinking

b Word salad

c Pressured speech

d Echolalia

e Thought blocking

147 A middle-aged woman with a known history of depression presents to her GP. During the consultation you observe she is tearful and withdrawn but she denies feeling low in mood or even crying. What term most appropriately describes such a phenomenon?

   a Agitation

   b Ambivalence

   c Alexithymia

   d Anxiety

   e Phobia

148 A patient with no known history of mental illness presents to his GP. He states that before falling asleep he sees an image of Christ at the end of his bed. What term most appropriately describes such a hallucination?

   a Somatic

   b Hypnopompic

   c Functional

   d Extracampine

   e Hypnagogic

149 A middle-aged gentleman with a known history of schizophrenia presents to his GP. He comments that he sees images of himself around the house and at work functioning in a similar way to him. What term most appropriately describes such a hallucination?

a Somatic

b Autoscopy

c Functional

d Extracampine

e Hypnagogic

150 A 32-year-old gentleman presents to his GP complaining of seeing images of his deceased father every morning as he awakes from sleep. What term most appropriately describes such a hallucination?

a Somatic

b Hypnopompic

c Functional

d Extracampine

e Hypnagogic

151 A middle-aged gentleman is referred for psychotherapy to help with his fear of spiders. The psychotherapist explains that he will be exposed to several spiders all at once. What term most appropriately describes this form of therapy?

a Systematic desensitization

b Flooding

c Response prevention

d Modelling

e Thought stopping

152 A patient with a known history of mental illness presents to his GP. During the consultation you enquire about how he has been feeling recently. You note that he answers the question eventually but discusses several different things prior to doing so. What term most appropriately describes such a phenomenon?

a Flight of ideas

b Circumstantiality

c Passing by the point

d Talking past the point

e Neologism

153   A patient with a known history of mental illness presents to his GP. During the consultation you note he repeats the word 'hello' several times. What term most appropriately describes such a phenomenon?

a   Passing by the point

b   Talking past the point

c   Palilalia

d   Logoclonia

e   Echolalia

154   The following are all true with regard to late onset schizophrenia EXCEPT:

a   The condition primarily affects males

b   The condition is associated with individuals aged 60 or over

c   Individuals demonstrate good premorbid intellectual functioning

d   Individuals demonstrate good premorbid occupational functioning

e   The condition is associated with organic brain dysfunction

155   The following are all true with regard to congenital schizophrenia EXCEPT:

a   The condition arises due to environmental factors

b   The condition primarily affects females

c   Long-term outcome is poor

d   The condition arises due to genetic factors

e   Individuals may demonstrate social impairment in childhood

156 The following are all true with regard to adult onset schizophrenia EXCEPT:

    a It is not associated with changes in mood

    b It may be associated with thought disorder

    c It may be associated with thought withdrawal

    d It may be associated with delusions

    e It may be associated with hallucinations

157 A middle-aged woman with a known history of anxiety is commenced on buspirone. The following are true with regard to buspirone EXCEPT:

    a It is administered orally

    b It is a partial agonist

    c It acts via GABA receptors

    d It is associated with nausea

    e It does not cause dependence

158 A patient with a known history of depression is commenced on mirtazapine. The following are all true with regard to mirtazapine EXCEPT:

    a It increases noradrenaline release

    b It acts as an agonist at alpha 2 adrenoceptors

    c It increases serotonin release

    d It is administered orally

    e It is associated with sedation

159 The following are all true with regard to reboxetine EXCEPT:

a It is useful in the treatment of depression

b It prevents the reuptake of noradrenaline

c It is administered orally

d It is associated with diarrhoea

e It is associated with urinary retention

160 The following are all true with regard to isocarboxazid EXCEPT:

a It is an example of a selective serotonin reuptake inhibitor

b It is administered orally

c It interacts dangerously with tricyclic antidepressants

d It is associated with hepatotoxicity

e It may cause weight gain

Extended matching questions

Theme: The Mental Health Act

a Section 2

b Section 3

c Section 4

d Section 5(2)

e Section 136

f Section 135

g Section 62

h Section 17

i Section 23

j Section 1

For each scenario described below, choose the single most appropriate answer from the above list of options. Each option may be used once, more than once or not at all.

1 A holding power for a maximum of 72 hours if a patient admitted informally threatens to leave hospital.

2 A section utilised for patients to be admitted as an emergency for assessment.

3 A patient found in a local shopping centre, threatening to harm herself and harm others.

4 A patient with a background history of paranoid schizophrenia being granted one hour unescorted leave from the hospital grounds daily.

5 A middle-aged woman presenting with a first-ever episode of auditory hallucinations; she has a known history of cannabis misuse.

Theme: Drugs

a Procyclidine

b Olanzapine

c Citalopram

d Lithium

e Paracetamol

f Moclobemide

g Venlafaxine

h Risperidone

i Clozapine

j Haloperidol

For each scenario described below, choose the single most appropriate answer from the above list of options. Each option may be used once, more than once or not at all.

1 A 32-year-old woman presents to her GP complaining of feeling low in mood, with poor sleep and appetite loss. She has recently lost her husband following a road traffic accident.

2 A 23-year-old woman presents with evidence of acute psychosis. She is admitted informally but begins to threaten staff and other patients.

3 A middle-aged woman presents claiming she is the best looking woman in England. During the consultation you note evidence of pressured speech and irritability. She begins to take off her clothes as you continue to take a history.

4   An agent that prevents the reuptake of noradrenaline and serotonin.

5   An agent commonly used to reduce the extrapyramidal side-effects of antipsychotic drugs.

Theme: Side-effects

a Olanzapine

b Haloperidol

c Lithium

d Carbamazepine

e Phenelzine

f ECT

g Fluoxetine

h Citalopram

i Clozapine

j Lorazepam

For each scenario described below, choose the single most appropriate answer from the above list of options. Each option may be used once, more than once or not at all.

1 An agent commonly associated with weight gain and hyperglycaemia.

   a

2 A drug known to cause a hypertensive crisis if taken with alcohol.

   e

3 Associated with headaches, confusion and memory loss.

   f

4 Associated with neutropenia and prolonged QT syndrome.

   i

5 A drug known to cause hypothyroidism and nephrotoxicity.

   c

Theme: Types of delusion

a Reference

b Grandeur

c Somatic

d Bizarre

e Nihilistic

f Doubles

g Self-accusation

h Poverty

i Querulant

j Erotomania

For each scenario described below, choose the single most appropriate answer from the above list of options. Each option may be used once, more than once or not at all.

1 A middle-aged gentleman stating that he is as great as the President of the United States and could do his job with his eyes closed.

    b

2 A middle-aged Turkish gentleman who believes he is going to be tortured by his neighbours.

    i (persecutory)

3 A 23-year-old woman who believes that the world is about to end.

    e

4 A 17-year-old teenager who believes that his ears control the broadcasting capability of BBC Radio One.

    c

5 A highly successful businessman who believes he only has enough money to purchase a slice of bread.

    h

Theme: Psychiatric disorders I

a Schizophrenia

b Depression

c Bipolar affective disorder

d Generalised anxiety disorder

e Anorexia nervosa

f Dementia

g Agoraphobia

h Bulimia nervosa

i Delirium

j Hypothyroidism

For each scenario described below, choose the single most appropriate answer from the above list of options. Each option may be used once, more than once or not at all.

1 A 23-year-old cannabis misuser experiencing voices of a threatening nature.

2 A middle-aged woman who presents elated and irritable in mood with pressured speech and thought disorder.

3 A chronic alcohol misuser who complains of seeing spiders two days after an alcoholic binge.

4 A 75-year-old woman who presents with a labile mood and difficulty in performing everyday tasks.

5 A 32-year-old woman who has recently been divorced presenting low in mood with poor appetite, reduced sleep and thoughts of self-harm.

Theme: Psychiatric disorders II

a Depression

b Bipolar affective disorder

c Cyclothymia

d Dysthymia

e Agoraphobia

f Panic disorder

g Generalised anxiety disorder

h Social phobia

i Paranoid personality disorder

j Histrionic personality disorder

For each scenario described below, choose the single most appropriate answer from the above list of options. Each option may be used once, more than once or not at all.

1 Associated with palpitations, shortness of breath and dizziness with no predisposing trigger factor.

   g

2 Associated with a fear of public speaking and eating in public places.

   h

3 Associated with a fear of leaving home and travelling on public transport.

   e

4 Associated with poor sleep and a feeling of worthlessness, but the ability to cope with the demands of everyday life.

   d

5 A disorder of mood associated with periods of mild depression and mild elation.

   c

Theme: Mental state examination

a   Psychomotor agitation

b   Thought withdrawal

c   Thought broadcast

d   Delusion

e   Hallucination

f   Illusion

g   Pressured speech

h   Insight

i   Mutism

j   Knight's move

For each scenario described below, choose the single most appropriate answer from the above list of options. Each option may be used once, more than once or not at all.

1   A patient complaining of seeing shadows of her former husband.

   e

2   A 23-year-old woman who is difficult to interrupt and has increased rate and quantity of speech.

   g

3   A chronic schizophrenic who presents acutely psychotic following non-compliance with medication. She feels she is well and that the medication is useless.

   h

4   A patient with known bipolar affective disorder who presents fol-lowing non-compliance with medication. She continues to pace around the ward and does star jumps on occasion.

   a

5   A middle-aged woman who believes she can communicate with birds in the trees by drawing on a piece of paper.

   d

Theme: Investigations

a Full blood count

b Liver function tests

c Thyroid function tests

d Serum prolactin

e Serum albumin

f Serum urea and electrolytes

g Chest X-ray

h Electrocardiogram

i Chest CT scan

j Echocardiogram

For each scenario described below, choose the single most appropriate answer from the above list of options. Each option may be used once, more than once or not at all.

1 A patient due to start clozapine following no improvement in her mental state with olanzapine or quetiapine.

2 A patient recently started on clozapine complaining of a sore throat and fever.

3 A patient due to start lithium following an episode of acute mania.

4 A patient on long-term lithium complaining of weight gain and cold intolerance.

5 A known schizophrenic patient currently on olanzapine complaining of reduced libido and gynaecomastia.

Theme: Mechanism of action of drugs

a Dopamine

b Histamine

c Serotonin

d Acetylcholine

e Noradrenaline

f Noradrenaline and serotonin

g GABA

h Monoamine oxidase type A

i Adrenaline

j Prolactin

For each scenario described below, choose the single most appropriate answer from the above list of options. Each option may be used once, more than once or not at all.

1 Imipramine can cause a dry mouth and blurred vision due to blockade of this neurotransmitter.

2 Olanzapine can cause a reduced libido and sperm count due to blockade of this neurotransmitter.

3 Lorazepam works by binding to benzodiazepine receptors linked to this receptor.

4 Olanzapine can cause postural hypotension and failure of ejaculation due to blockade of this neurotransmitter.

5 Antipsychotics can be associated with sedation due to blockade of this neurotransmitter.

Theme: Substance misuse

a Alcohol

b Cocaine

c Paracetamol

d Heroin

e Cannabis

f Benzodiazepines

g Ecstasy

h Caffeine

i Solvents

j Amphetamines

For each scenario described below, choose the single most appropriate answer from the above list of options. Each option may be used once, more than once or not at all.

1 A substance commonly associated with pin-point pupils and a tremor.

2 A substance commonly taken in overdose and known to affect the liver.

3 A substance associated with auditory or visual hallucinations as well as an increased appetite.

4 A substance associated with thiamine deficiency following long-term misuse.

5 A substance commonly associated with myocardial ischaemia and subsequent infarction.

Answers

Single best answer

1   d

Schneider's first rank symptoms include auditory hallucinations, thought insertion, thought withdrawal, thought broadcast, delusional perception, made feelings and somatic passivity.

2   c

Paranoid schizophrenia is characterised by the following symptoms: delusions of persecution, delusions of reference, delusions of bodily change, delusions of jealously and auditory hallucinations.

3   b

Catatonic schizophrenia is characterised by motor immobility, excessive motor activity, peculiar voluntary movements or evidence of negativism.

4   e

Alcohol misuse is not an associated risk factor. Additional risk factors include genetic factors, certain personality types and prenatal complications.

5   d

This patient has evidence of auditory hallucinations as well as delusions of persecution and hence is suffering from schizophrenia. The age of onset of schizophrenia is commonly between 15 and 45 years.

6   c

This patient has evidence of delusional beliefs and strong spiritualistic preoccupations. The most likely working diagnosis is schizophrenia and hence olanzapine would be the drug of choice.

7   e

This patient has strong delusional beliefs that have been sparked following non-compliance with her oral medication. She has limited insight and feels the medication does not help. In these situations the risk of recommencing oral medication would mean that she is likely to not comply following discharge from hospital and hence a depot medication would be more suitable.

8   c

Erotomania is where an individual holds a strong belief that someone of a higher status is in love with them.

9   c

Suicide is more common in spring and early summer.

10   a

Deliberate self-harm is most commonly seen between the ages of 15 and 25.

11   d

A Section 5(2) can be utilised as a holding power for 72 hours if a patient threatens to leave hospital having been admitted initially as an informal patient, particularly when there is evidence of mental state deterioration or a risk to either themselves or others.

12   c

Following haloperidol the patient has developed extra pyramidal side-effects. Procyclidine is an anti muscarinic agent, which is a useful form of treatment.

13   a

This patient has biological features of depression and hence is likely to be experiencing a reduced libido.

14   d

Pressured speech is most likely a feature of acute mania as opposed to depression.

15   a

Weight loss is classically a feature of a major depressive episode. Additional features include low mood, anhedonia, insomnia or hyper-somnia, psychomotor agitation, energy loss, poor concentration, suicidal ideation and feelings of worthlessness or guilt.

16   b

Depression is most commonly associated around the mid to late 30s.

17   e

This patient has classical biological features of depression. A selective serotonin reuptake inhibitor such as citalopram is the first-line treatment in such cases.

18   e

This is certainly a concerning case. The patient is notably depressed and is refusing oral medication and nutritional support. As a result she has become hypotensive and is failing to pass urine. In such cases, ECT is the treatment of choice, particularly as she has little insight into her illness and wants to end her life.

19   d

This patient has clear features of acute mania and hence is likely to demonstrate evidence of psychomotor agitation as opposed to retardation.

20   c

Evidence to suggest such a diagnosis is based on her mental state assessment of an elated mood, pressured speech and psychomotor agitation.

21   c

In cases of bipolar affective disorder and an acute manic presentation, research has demonstrated that an antipsychotic such as olanzapine.is often first-line treatment.

22   d

This patient is notably psychotic and hence olanzapine would be the treatment of choice.

23   a

This case demonstrates evidence of acute psychosis and possible catatonic schizophrenia. Hence an antipsychotic such as amisulpride would be the first line management.

24   a

Olanzapine is an antipsychotic agent and mainly works via blockade of dopamine receptors, but also serotonin receptors.

25   d

This patient is acutely psychotic. He is notably deluded and experiencing auditory hallucinations. Research suggests that clozapine is the next drug of choice in these cases where a trial of at least two antipsychotics for at least a six-week period each demonstrates no real improvement in mental state.

26   e

Antipsychotics are likely to cause constipation due to antimuscarinic effects.

27   d

Antipsychotics have anticholinergic effects, which lead to a dry mouth, blurred vision, urinary retention and constipation.

28   b

Antipsychotics such as risperidone have antidopaminergic effects, which result in elevated prolactin and subsequent galactorrhoea, gynaecomastia, menstrual irregularities and reduced libido.

29   b

Antipsychotics through their antidopaminergic action result in extrapyramidal side-effects, notably parkinsonism, dystonias, akathisia and tardive dyskinesia.

30   b

This patient is demonstrating evidence of neuroleptic malignant syndrome, a side-effect of antipsychotic medication. Clinical features include hyperthermia, a fluctuating conscious level, tachycardia, muscular rigidity and urinary incontinence.

31   d

This patient is suffering from neuroleptic malignant syndrome. Common blood abnormalities include a raised creatine phosphokinase, elevated white cell count and deranged liver function.

32   a

Clozapine has been shown to cause QT prolongation and tachyarrhythmias. A baseline ECG is needed to exclude pre-existing cardiac disease prior to commencement.

33   c

Clozapine has been shown to cause neutropenia and hence a full blood count is needed at least once weekly to ensure no evidence of such an occurrence.

34   e

This patient has evidence of acute psychosis. She has a medical history of cardiac disease and dementia. Current guidelines state that atypical antipsychotics such as risperidone or olanzapine should be avoided in patients with dementia due to an increased risk of cerebrovascular events. And hence haloperidol, a typical antipsychotic, would be the drug of choice.

35   a

Atypical antipsychotics commonly cause weight gain.

36   d

Lithium is associated with hyper or hypothyroidism and nephrotoxicity. Liver function tests are not necessary with regard to lithium monitoring.

37   d

Lithium is known to cause weight gain.

38   c

Common side-effects of lithium include nausea, a metallic taste, a dry mouth, diarrhoea, tremor and polyuria.

39   e

Lithium levels should be monitored, ideally 8–12 hours post-dose.

40   c

The most appropriate therapeutic plasma range of lithium is between 0.4–1.0 mmol/L.

41   c

Signs of lithium toxicity include ataxia, blurred vision, tinnitus, diarrhoea and muscle weakness.

42   e

Carbamazepine is known to cause renal and hepatic impairment. It is also associated with blood dyscrasias and bone marrow suppression.

43   b

Carbamazepine has been associated with ocular side-effects such as cortical lens opacities and conjunctivitis.

44   d

Tricyclic antidepressants inhibit the reuptake of noradrenaline and serotonin.

45   a

Imipramine is an example of a tricyclic antidepressant. Common ECG changes include T wave flattening, QT interval prolongation and ST depression.

46   b

Tricyclic antidepressants such as imipramine are associated with blurred vision, a dry mouth, nausea, a blackened tongue, arrhythmias, urinary retention, constipation and weight gain.

47   a

Venlafaxine is an example of a selective noradrenaline and serotonin reuptake inhibitor.

48 d

Imipramine is a tricyclic antidepressant. Such drugs are associated with agranulocytosis, leukopenia, eosinophilia and thrombocytopenia.

49 a

Phenelzine is a monoamine oxidase inhibitor. Such drugs are known to cause a hypertensive crisis if taken with tyramine containing foods such as cheese, alcohol, meat and fish.

50 a

This patient has developed a hypertensive crisis. Monoamine oxidase inhibitors such as phenelzine have been found to induce such a crisis with sympathomimetic amines such as those found in cough mixtures and nasal decongestants.

51 d

This patient has developed a hypertensive crisis following phenelzine and alcohol misuse. Reversible inhibitors of monoamine oxidase A such as moclobemide do not classically cause such a reaction with tyramine containing products.

52 c

Lorazepam is a short acting benzodiazepine. Other examples include lormetazepam and temazepam.

53 c

Diazepam is a benzodiazepine. Their mode of action involves binding to GABA receptors in combination with benzodiazepine receptors and chloride channels.

54 d

Benzodiazepines such as diazepam can result in a withdrawal syndrome characterised by low mood, depersonalisation, derealisation, tinnitus, appetite loss and seizures if stopped suddenly.

55 e

The main side-effects of ECT include a headache, confusion and memory loss.

56 e

The main contraindications of ECT include raised intracranial pressure, cardiac and respiratory disease.

57 b

Personalisation is whereby negative events are personalised to oneself leading to guilt.

58 b

This patient is acutely psychotic. Olanzapine is the drug of choice in pregnancy.

59 d

The most likely timeframe for the occurrence of postnatal depression is between two and six weeks postpartum.

60 c

The International Classification of Diseases (ICD-10) criterion for body weight in anorexia nervosa is that it is maintained at least 15% below expected.

61   a

Constipation is classically seen in anorexia nervosa.

62   c

Hypokalaemia is commonly seen due to vomiting. Additional abnormalities include anaemia, leukopenia, thrombocytopenia, hyper-cholesterolaemia and hypomagnesaemia.

63   a

ST depression is commonly seen in anorexia nervosa.

64   c

Russell's sign refers to the presence of calluses on the dorsum of the hand in patients who use their fingers to stimulate the gag reflex.

65   b

High-dose antidepressant medication has been shown to be effective in severe cases of bulimia.

66   b

Ambitendency is the term used to describe a series of tentative incomplete movements made when expected to carry out a voluntary action.

67   d

Waxy flexibility is where movement of the individual's body results in a feeling of plastic resistance and then subsequent preservation of the final posture.

68 e

Classical features of delirium following alcohol withdrawal. Prodromal symptoms include a hypersensitivity to light and sound. Delirium itself is characterised by agitation, hallucinations and impaired memory.

69 b

Metabolic causes of delirium include hepatic, renal, respiratory and cardiac failure. Additional causes include thiamine, nicotinic acid, folate and vitamin B12 deficiency.

70 b

Classical presentation of dementia. Dementia typically presents from the age of 60 onwards and comprises features such as delusional beliefs, disorientation in time, place and person, as well as comprehension and language impairment.

71 b

Alzheimer's disease is the commonest cause of dementia in the over 65 age range.

72 e

Accumulation of beta amyloid protein is seen in Alzheimer's disease.

73 a

Donepezil, a reversible acetylcholinesterase inhibitor, has been shown to be effective in the treatment of Alzheimer's disease.

74 d

Memantine is a NMDA receptor antagonist used in the treatment of Alzheimer's disease.

75   e

Rivastigmine is a reversible non-competitive inhibitor of acetyl-cholinesterase.

76   e

Lewy body dementia is characterised by cognitive impairment, parkinsonism and visual hallucinations.

77   b

Frontotemporal dementia is characterised by inattention, reduced speech, apathy, withdrawal and akinesia.

78   c

Taking into account her past medical history, the most likely diagnosis is vascular dementia.

79   d

Korsakov's syndrome is an impairment of recent memory with preservation of immediate recall. It is commonly seen in chronic alcohol misusers.

80   e

Korsakov's syndrome in alcoholics is due to thiamine deficiency.

81   a

Frontal lobe damage is characterised by personality changes in the main, with an elevated mood, irritability and reduced social and ethical control.

82 b

Temporal lobe damage is characterised mainly by sensory aphasia, alexia and agraphia.

83 d

This patient is suffering from Gerstmann's syndrome, which is characterised by dyscalculia, agraphia, finger agnosia and right to left disorientation.

84 d

Gerstmann's syndrome is seen in parietal lobe damage.

85 b

This patient has evidence of occipital lobe damage, more specifically a non-dominant lesion. This is characterised by visuospatial agnosia, prosopagnosia, metamorphopsia and visual hallucinations.

86 c

Such features are seen in occipital lobe damage, more specifically a non-dominant lesion.

87 e

Thalamic lesions often cause hyperalgesia to painful stimuli.

88 a

Such a section is primarily for assessment purposes and lasts for a total of 28 days.

89 e

Section 2 of the Mental Health Act lasts for a total of 28 days.

90   b

Section 2 of the Mental Health Act is primarily for assessment purposes.

91   c

Two medical practitioners are required for a Section 2 recommendation.

92   e

Following a placement under Section 2 of the Mental Health Act, patients have 14 days with which to appeal.

93   d

Section 136 of the Mental Health Act is used by police to bring an individual from a public place to a place of safety for assessment purposes.

94   b

This patient is acutely psychotic with strong delusional beliefs following non-compliance with medication. Section 3 of the Mental Health Act would be the most appropriate section here to enable an admission for treatment purposes.

95   e

Section 3 of the Mental Health Act lasts a total of six months.

96   c

The patient's nearest relative or hospital manager can appeal such a decision.

97   c

Section 4 allows for emergency admission for assessment purposes.

98   e

Section 4 of the Mental Health Act can last a total of 72 hours.

99   a

Agoraphobia is an anxiety-causing phobia, which is associated with fear of leaving home, crowds and public places.

100   e

This patient has evidence of agoraphobia, which is most appropriately managed with behavioural therapy.

101   b

Classical features of social phobia whereby people are fearful of being scrutinised in groups leading to avoidance of social situations.

102   e

Behavioural therapy is the treatment of choice for social phobia.

103   d

Classical features of a panic disorder. Such disorders are characterised by palpitations, chest pain, dizziness, sweating, depersonalisation, derealisation and a fear of dying.

104   d

This patient is suffering from a panic disorder, which is most appropriately managed with antidepressants such as imipramine.

105   b

Generalised anxiety disorder is often characterised by diarrhoea and not constipation.

106   d

This patient is suffering from generalised anxiety disorder. If there is no improvement of symptoms with antidepressants or anxiolytics research suggests the use of beta blockers and behavioural therapy.

107   d

Obsessive compulsive disorder is characterised by obsessional thoughts and compulsive acts, such as hand washing in this particular example.

108   b

Antidepressants, commonly selective serotonin reuptake inhibitors, are first-line management in the treatment of obsessive compulsive disorder.

109   d

Post-traumatic stress disorder is characterised by a delayed response to a stressful or catastrophic event. Patients experience flashbacks, emotional blunting and anhedonia.

110   b

Adjustment disorder is whereby patients experience a depressive or anxiety-type reaction following a significant life change or event.

111   b

Ganser's syndrome is a conversion disorder characterised by the giving of approximate answers.

112   b

Such a syndrome is characterised by a preoccupation of having one or more serious physical disorders.

113   b

Paranoid personality disorder is characterised by an excessive sensitivity to setbacks with suspicion and a preoccupation with unsubstantiated explanations of events.

114   d

A histrionic personality disorder is characterised by excessive emotion, attention seeking, self-dramatisation and over concern with physical attractiveness. Excitement is continually sought, as is the appreciation of others.

115   b

Such a disorder is characterised by a dependent and submissive behaviour. Such individuals feel helpless, have difficulty in initiating projects and often require a high level of reassurance.

116   b

Classical presentation of an alcoholic withdrawal, which may also be complicated by delirium or convulsions.

117   c

Dependence is classically associated with the use of a particular substance on a continuous or periodic basis and has a higher priority than other behaviours previously.

118   a

Tolerance is where the desired central nervous system effects of a particular substance diminish with repeated usage so that increasing doses are needed to achieve the required effect.

119   d

Chronic alcohol misuse is associated with a macrocytic anaemia due to folate and B12 deficiency.

120   c

Wernicke's encephalopathy is associated with opthalmoplegia, nystagmus, ataxia, altered consciousness and peripheral neuropathy.

121   e

Alcohol dependency is classically associated with a narrowing of the drinking repertoire.

122   d

Hypomania is a predisposing disorder to alcohol dependency.

123   a

Disulfiram results in facial flushing, headaches, tachycardias, palpitations and nausea if taken in conjunction with alcohol.

124   b

Acetaldehyde accumulation is primarily responsible for such side-effects with disulfiram and alcohol intake.

125   a

Pinpoint pupils are classical of opioid misuse such as heroin.

126   e

Cannabis misuse results in strong delusional beliefs, social withdrawal, depersonalisation, derealisation and an increased appetite.

127   a

Cocaine misuse has been strongly associated with myocardial ischaemia and subsequent infarction.

128   b

MDMA or Ecstasy is a hallucinogen associated with hallucinations, depersonalisation and derealisation. Physical effects include dilated pupils, tachycardia, palpitations, sweating and blurred vision.

129   c

Alzheimer's disease is characterised by cerebral atrophy and not pseudodementia.

130   d

Alzheimer's disease is characterised by slow wave activity on the EEG. A normal EEG is typically seen in pseudodementia.

131   a

Attention deficit hyperactivity disorder is characterised by impaired attention and over activity. Associated features include disinhibition in social relationships, recklessness and the impulsive defying of rules.

132   c

Conduct disorder is characterised by a repetitive and persistent pattern of aggressive or defiant conduct. It is characterised by aggression to people or animals, destruction of property, theft and serious rule violation.

133   e

Conduct disorder is classically managed by psychotherapy.

134   b

This patient is suffering from functional enuresis, which is attributed to genetic factors in 70% of cases.

135   a

Such drugs have proven to be beneficial in cases of enuresis due to their antimuscarinic action.

136   b

Echopraxia is defined as the automatic imitation of another person's movements.

137   b

Such a term describes a person's speech, which is fluent and rambling in nature.

138   d

A neologism is a newly made up word or a commonly used word that is used in a special way.

139   c

Such a delusion is a belief pertaining to the functioning of one's body part or parts.

140   a

Thought alienation is a term used to describe an individual's belief that their thoughts are under the control of an outside group or organisation.

141   d

A delusion whereby an individual has an exaggerated belief of their own power or importance.

142   b

A classic description of word salad or schizophasia associated with an incoherent and incomprehensible mixture of words and phrases.

143   e

Thought blocking is essentially an abrupt interruption in an individual's thought process and is associated with no recall of what was being discussed.

144   a

A disorder of speech characterised by odd associations between ideas and ultimately poor speech continuity.

145   c

A classic description of flight of ideas associated with sudden changes between topics with no obvious focus.

146   d

A classic description of echolalia.

147   c

A disorder whereby an individual is unaware or unable to describe their true feelings or emotions.

148   e

A classic description of such a form of hallucination.

149   b

A classic description of such a hallucination.

150   b

Such a hallucination may be auditory in nature as well.

151   b

Such a form of therapy is often repeated several times until the anxiety is relieved.

152   b

Such a speech disorder is associated with discussion of several unnecessary details prior to reaching the final answer or thought.

153   c

A classic description of such a phenomenon.

154   a

Late onset schizophrenia primarily affects females.

155   b

Congenital schizophrenia primarily affects males.

156   a

Adult onset schizophrenia is often associated with changes in mood.

157   c

Buspirone acts via serotonin receptors, specifically type 1A.

158   b

Mirtazapine is an antagonist at alpha 2 adrenoceptors.

159   d

Reboxetine is associated with constipation. Additional side-effects include increased sweating and insomnia.

160   a

Isocarboxazid is an example of a monoamine oxidase inhibitor.

Extended matching questions

Theme: The Mental Health Act

1   d

Such a section can only be utilised by the doctor in charge of the patient in question.

2   c

Such a section lasts for a maximum of 72 hours.

3   e

A section utilised by the police, which allows a patient to be brought to a place of safety for assessment. It lasts for a maximum of 72 hours.

4   h

Such a section is authorised by the responsible medical officer allocated to the patient and is often subject to conditions.

5   a

This section is an assessment section and lasts for a maximum of 28 days.

Theme: Drugs

1   c

This patient has notable features of depression. Selective serotonin reuptake inhibitors are the first-line treatment for depression.

2   j

Haloperidol is an antipsychotic and can be used for rapid tranquilisation purposes in cases of patient agitation or distress.

3   b

This patient is acutely manic. Current guidelines recommend the use of antipsychotics such as olanzapine for the treatment of acute mania.

4   g

Venlafaxine is an antidepressant and may cause hypertension at high doses.

5   a

Such an agent is an antimuscarinic and can be administered orally, intramuscularly or intravenously.

Theme: Side-effects

1 a

Additional side-effects include gynaecomastia, galactorrhoea, parkinsonism, urinary retention, blurred vision and constipation.

2 e

Such an agent commonly induces an elevated blood pressure in association with tyramine containing foods such as alcohol, cheese, meat and fish.

3 f

Common side-effects of ECT.

4 i

Clozapine is associated with neutropenia and cardiovascular complications such as prolonged QT syndrome. Regular blood monitoring and a baseline ECG is needed prior to starting such medication.

5 c

Lithium is also associated with hyperthyroidism and cardiovascular abnormalities.

Theme: Types of delusion

1   b

A classical description of a delusion of grandeur whereby an individual has an exaggerated belief of their own power or importance.

2   i

Also commonly referred to as a persecutory delusion.

3   e

Such a delusion describes a belief whereby oneself or the world does not exist or is about to cease to exist.

4   c

A belief pertaining to the functioning of one's body part or parts.

5   h

Classical description of a delusion of poverty.

Theme: Psychiatric disorders I

1   a

Additional features may include visual hallucinations, formal thought disorder or thought interference.

2   c

A classical description of bipolar affective disorder. Additional features may include poor sleep, psychomotor agitation and increased sexual promiscuity.

3   i

Prodromal symptoms may include an increased sensitivity to sound or light.

4   f

This patient is likely to be suffering from Alzheimer's disease, the most common form of dementia.

5   b

Classical biological features of depression. Additional features may include reduced energy levels and concentration.

Theme: Psychiatric disorders II

1   g

Such individuals may also experience a dry mouth, epigastric pain, muscle tension and urinary frequency.

2   h

Management of such a condition is through behavioural therapy.

3   e

This disorder is commonly seen in the mid to late 20s. The treatment of choice is behavioural therapy.

4   d

This disorder is commonly seen in females. Management involves treatment with antidepressants, psychotherapy or cognitive behavioural therapy.

5   c

Treatment classically involves the use of lithium or psychotherapy.

Theme: Mental state examination

1   e

A false sensory perception occurring in the absence of a real external stimulus.

2   g

Classical description of pressured speech, commonly seen in an acute manic episode.

3   h

This patient has limited insight and is likely to be a difficult case to manage from a compliance point of view.

4   a

Excessive motor activity associated with a feeling of inner tension.

5   d

A fixed false personal belief that is sustained in spite of what others believe or evidence to the contrary.

Theme: Investigations

1   h

Clozapine has been associated with prolonged QT syndrome and tachyarrhythmias. A baseline ECG is always required to rule out pre-existing cardiac disease.

2   a

Clozapine is known to cause neutropenia and hence a weekly full blood count is needed during treatment on this medication.

3   f

Prior to commencement of lithium, one must check the serum urea and electrolytes as the drug is excreted by the kidneys and is highly nephrotoxic. Long-term lithium use requires monitoring of thyroid function as the drug can cause hyper or hypothyroidism.

4   c

This patient has developed hypothyroidism as a result of long-term lithium use.

5   d

Antipsychotics such as olanzapine cause dopamine blockade and subsequent hyperprolactinaemia. This, in turn, causes galactorrhoea, gynaecomastia, menstrual disturbances, reduced libido and a reduced sperm count.

Theme: Mechanism of action of drugs

1   d

Additional symptoms may include urinary retention and constipation.

2   a

This is primarily due to an elevated prolactin as a result of dopamine blockade.

3   g

The end result is a complex involving GABA, a benzodiazepine receptor and a chloride channel.

4   i

Classically seen with all antipsychotics.

5   b

Classically seen with all antipsychotics, not just olanzapine.

Theme: Substance misuse

1   d

Additional features may include erectile dysfunction and constipation.

2   c

Paracetamol is commonly taken in overdose as it is easily available. Treatment involves the use of N-acetylcysteine or NAC.

3   e

Additional features may include a dry mouth, cough and infection of the conjunctiva.

4   a

Such deficiency results in Wernicke's encephalopathy. Features of this disorder include nystagmus, ophthalmoplegia, ataxia and peripheral neuropathy.

5   b

Cocaine is commonly associated with such a complication as a result of coronary artery spasm. Additional cardiac complications include left ventricular hypertrophy, arrhythmias, heart failure and myocarditis.

Index

Page numbers to questions (Q) and answers (A) are given in the following format, Q/A